How To Lose Weight Without Stress

14 recommendations for fit, healthier
and obese free living

Jason Higginss

Table of Contents

12. Create a strategy.
13. Seek out social services
14. Keep a positive attitude

Introduction

Despite the abundance of "fad" diets available, a nutritious diet combined with a balanced lifestyle is the key to better weight control and a healthy living.

Among other serious health problems, being overweight increases the risk of heart disease, hypertension, and type 2 diabetes.
Crash diets are not a long-term solution, regardless of any advantages that its proponents may assert. For safe, long-term weight loss, it is imperative to make tiny but beneficial lifestyle changes.
A few doable actions can help people lose weight and keep it off. These are some of the test and trusted tips and guidelines that could help you live obese free.

1.Take charge of the area where you eat.

Take charge of your eating environment by deciding what, when, and how much you eat, as well as what items you always have on hand.

At home, prepare your own food. This gives you control over the components and amount of the food. Generally speaking, home-cooked food has fewer calories, sugar, and fat grams per serving than food from restaurants or packaged products.

Cut back on how much you serve yourself. Use small plates, glasses, and dishes to make your food look larger. Eat straight out of large dishes or food containers to prevent making it more difficult to track how much you've eaten.

Eat ahead of time. Studies show that consuming more of your daily caloric intake at breakfast and less at dinner will help you lose more weight. You may boost your metabolism, decrease hunger pangs, and burn off more calories throughout the day by eating a larger, healthier breakfast.

Try to eat dinner early, and then fast till breakfast the next morning. Eating solely during times of intense activity and taking long pauses from food digestion may help with weight loss.

Plan ahead for your meals and snacks. Plastic containers or bags can be used to produce your own small snacks. By keeping a schedule and eating only when you are truly hungry, you can avoid overindulging in food.

Consume more water. Since many times hunger and thirst are confused, drinking water can help you reduce your calorie intake.

Limit how many delicious foods you have in your house. If you have someone in your kitchen who isn't on a diet, keep the tempting meals covered.

2. Eat a diverse range of colorful, nutrient-rich meals.

Nutritious meals and snacks should form the cornerstone of a person's diet. A simple way to create a meal plan is to make sure that each meal contains 50% fruit and vegetables, 25% whole grains, and 25% protein. In all, 25–30 grams of fiber should be ingested.

Eliminate trans fats from your diet and limit your intake of saturated fats, which are closely linked to the risk of coronary heart disease.

People may choose to consume unsaturated fats such as monounsaturated fatty acids (MUFA) and polyunsaturated fatty acids (PUFA) as an alternative.

The following foods are nutrient-dense and often contain a lot of nutrients:
fresh fruits and vegetables

fish, whole grains including brown rice and oats, lentils, seeds, and nuts

Products that you need not to eat consist of:

consuming processed meats with added sugar, butter, or oils, or rich red meats

baked goods

bagels

White bread.

cooked dinners

Eliminating specific foods from the diet might occasionally leave a person deficient in vital vitamins and minerals. A nutritionist, dietician, or other medical expert can advise someone who is on a weight loss program on how to make sure they are obtaining enough nutrients.

3. Keep a diet and weight journal.

Self-monitoring is essential to successful weight loss. People can use a paper notebook, mobile app, or specialized website to track every food item they eat each day. Maintaining a weekly weight record is another method they could use to monitor their progress.

If a person can track their progress in little steps and observe bodily changes, they have a considerably higher chance of sticking with a weight loss program.

People can also keep an eye on their body mass index (BMI) with a BMI calculator.

Despite the abundance of "fad" diets available, a healthy lifestyle is centered around a balanced diet.

Being overweight increases the likelihood of serious health problems, including heart disease, hypertension, and diabetes.

4. Examine nutrition labels.

Establishing the habit of turning your packages over will save you calories, money, and time.

The food labels provide you a realistic picture of what's in your food.

When attempting a healthy weight loss plan, it's critical to remember that calories count, so pay close attention to product labels.

For your meals to be nutritionally valuable, you must eat a balanced diet free of added sugars, sodium, and saturated fat.

5. Make regular use of exercise and physical activity.

Studies have indicated that regular exercise can aid with weight loss.

To keep one's physical and mental health in check, regular exercise is essential. Sometimes the key to successful weight loss is to increase physical activity frequency in a controlled and intentional manner.

Walking briskly is one form of moderate-to-intense exercise that is advised for one hour per day. Should achieving an hour daily prove unattainable, the Mayo Clinic recommends attempting to obtain a minimum of 150 minutes each week.

It's advisable for those who don't often exercise to progressively increase their exercise volume and intensity. The best way to guarantee that they make time for regular exercise is to ensure that regular exercise becomes a part of their lifestyle.

Keeping note of one's physical activity may have similar psychological benefits to weight loss as does journaling meals. Once a user logs their food consumption and exercise, a number of free smartphone apps are available to track their calorie balance.

For those who are new to exercising, the following activities can help them get more exercise if the idea of a full workout sounds daunting:
•use the stairs
•leaf raking
•dog walks
•gardening
•dancing
•playing outside games, and parking further away from a building entrance

People who are not at high risk for coronary heart disease are probably not going to need a medical evaluation before beginning an exercise program.

6. Get adequate sleep.

A healthy sleep schedule in addition to food and activity modifications may aid in weight loss.

A study found that people who regularly sleep for less than 7 hours are more likely to develop obesity and a higher body mass index than people who consistently slept for more than 7 hours.

In addition, hormones that control hunger and appetite may be altered by sleep deprivation.

Try to get 7 hours or more each night.As a general rule of thumb, trust a reliable source for restful sleep.

7. Get rid of liquid calories

Consuming tea, juice, sugar-filled sodas, or alcoholic beverages can add up to hundreds of calories every day. Since they increase energy content without enhancing nutrition, they are known as "empty calories".

Unless they are replacing meals with smoothies, a person should aim to keep their intake to no more than water, unsweetened tea, and coffee. You can flavor water by adding a squeeze of fresh lemon or orange.

Never mistake thirst for hunger. Between planned meals, a glass of water can often satisfy one's appetite.

8. Follow a Mediterranean diet and lifestyle

A diet rich in fresh fruits and vegetables, nuts, fish, olive oil, healthy fats, and carbs with little intake of meat and cheese is the foundation of the Mediterranean diet. The Mediterranean diet is more than just a set of recipes, though. Participating in frequent physical activity and eating meals with friends are also crucial components.

Whatever weight loss strategy you decide on, it's imperative to stay motivated and avoid common dieting pitfalls like emotional eating.

Lessen the emotional food you eat.

We don't always eat to satisfy our hunger. All too often, when we're anxious or upset, we resort to food, which can wreck any diet and result in weight gain. Do you eat when you're bored, lonely, or nervous? After a long day, do you relax with a snack in front of the TV? Comprehending the emotional eating triggers that you can steer clear of might significantly influence your efforts to lose weight. During mealtime, if you're bored or lonely, reach out to people rather than the fridge. Go for a stroll with your dog, make a call to a buddy who makes you laugh, or visit any public place where people congregate, like a park or library.

Try finding better techniques to de-stress if you're stressed. You could benefit from yoga, meditation, or a hot bath.

Do you lack energy? Seek out more midafternoon stimulants. Think about napping for a little while or taking a block walk.

9. Monitor amounts and calculate serving sizes

Any meal, even low-calorie vegetables, can cause weight gain if consumed in excess.

Therefore, customers should avoid eating food directly from the package or estimating portion sizes. Cups for measuring and serving sizes are useful tools. Assumptions raise the possibility of overeating and ingesting more food than is required.

The following size comparisons can be useful in monitoring portion sizes when dining out:

Half a cup is equal to a golf ball.

A tennis ball is equal to a half-cup.

One cup equals a baseball.

One ounce (oz) is equal to a loose handful of nuts.

A single die is equal to one tsp.

A tablespoon is a thumb tip.

Three ounces of meat is equal to a deck of cards.

A single DVD slice.

These measures are not exact, but they can help someone manage their food intake when the proper tools are unavailable.

10. Eat mindfully

Mindful eating, or being aware of what, when, how, where, and why one eats, has many benefits for many people.

Making better food choices is closely correlated with increased bodily awareness.

Aware eaters concentrate on the flavor of their meal in addition to attempting to eat more slowly and relish it. It takes the body 20 minutes to process all of the fullness signs after a meal.

It's important to focus on feeling satisfied rather than full after eating, and remember that not all "all natural" or low-fat items are necessarily good choices.

Before choosing a meal, people could also consider the following questions:
For the price of calories, is it a good "value"?

Will it satisfy me?
Are they healthy ingredients?
How much sodium and fat is in it, if it has a label?

11. Management of cues and stimuli

Overindulgent eating may be encouraged by a variety of social and environmental factors. For example, some people find that watching TV increases their tendency to overeat. Giving someone a bowl of candy without starting to nibble oneself is a challenge for some people.

By being aware of the things that could lead someone to crave empty calories, people can devise strategies to alter their daily routine to reduce these triggers.

12. Create a strategy.

Creating well-organized meal planning and stocking your kitchen with low-calorie foods will help you lose weight more quickly.

Eliminate processed and junk food from the kitchen and make sure you always have the ingredients on hand for easy, nutritious meals if you're trying to lose weight or keep it off. Eating that is careless, rushed, and unplanned can be prevented by doing this.

Organizing meals ahead of time before going to events or restaurants can also help the process.

13. Seek out social services

Social support plays a major role in maintaining motivation.
A good weight loss program requires you to accept the assistance of those you love.

Some will like to invite friends or family to join them, while others would like to share their progress via social media.
Other resources that could be useful are:
a companion, fitness centers, social networks that are encouraging, individual counseling, or workplace programs for employees 10. Remain positive.

Because weight loss is a gradual process, one may get discouraged if the pounds do not drop off as soon as they had thought.

There will be days when sticking to a weight loss or maintenance program is more challenging than others. A participant in a weight-loss program needs to remain persistent and not give up when it seems too difficult to make behavioral adjustments.

Social support has a major role in helping people stay motivated.
A weight loss program that works requires you to accept the assistance of the people you care about.

14. Keep a positive attitude

Since losing weight is a gradual process, one may get discouraged if the weight does not drop off as soon as they had intended.

There will be days when sticking to a weight loss or maintenance program is more challenging than others. The participant in a weight-loss program needs to be persistent and not give up when it seems too difficult to make behavioral changes.

Some may need to reset their goals in order to make adjustments to their exercise routine or their total caloric intake.

Remaining optimistic and tenaciously striving to surmount hindrances to successful weight loss are essential.

Gaining physical fitness

Without following a diet plan like Atkins or Slimming World, people can still lose weight. In order to achieve an energy imbalance, the focus should instead be on reducing calorie intake and increasing physical activity.

Weight loss results from a reduction in total calories consumed rather than from altering the proportions of fat, protein, and carbs in the diet.

To start reaping the health benefits, a 5- to 10-percent reduction in body weight over a 6-month period is a reasonable weight loss aim.

Most individuals can accomplish this goal by reducing their daily calorie consumption to 1,600–1,000 calories.

You cannot get enough nutrients for the full day with less than 1,000 calories per day.

Because people prefer to eat less energy when they are lighter, after six months of dieting, the rate of weight loss often slows down and body weight typically stabilizes. Following a weight maintenance program that incorporates regular exercise and good eating practices can help avoid the regain of lost weight.

Prescription: weight-loss medications may be helpful for those with a BMI of 30 or above who do not have any obesity-related health problems. Those with BMIs of 27 or above due to obesity may also benefit from these.

I'm summary,

The time to take the first step toward better future and fitter body is now.Find out how your mind can influence your weight loss journey. You goal to fitness should be how you like in your body.

Follow these above principles consistently and you will achieve your desired results.

Thank you for reading